HOLISTIC APPROACHES TO PREVENTING AND MANAGING ALZHEIMERS DISEASE

Comprehensive Guide to Holistic Strategies for Alzheimer's Prevention and Management

DR. CHRIS FRIEDRICH

Disclaimer

This book on Herbal Remedies is intended solely for informational and educational purposes.

The content provided within this book is based on general knowledge and should not be considered as professional advice. The author is not a licensed medical professional, and the information presented here is not intended to diagnose, treat, cure, or prevent any disease.

Readers are advised to consult with qualified healthcare professionals before initiating any herbal remedies or making changes to their existing health regimen. The author and publisher disclaim any responsibility for any adverse effects or consequences resulting from the use of information contained in this book.

It's important to note that the content of this book is not endorsed by any specific platform or affiliated with any product or service.

The author does not receive any compensation or benefits from the promotion of specific herbal products or brands.

Readers should exercise their discretion and judgment when applying the information from this book, and they are encouraged to conduct further research and seek guidance from healthcare professionals to make informed decisions about their health and well-being.

A thorough examination of the disease, including its definition, characteristics, causes, and stages, as well as a critical evaluation of current treatment approaches, are provided in Chapter 1 of the book, which also lays the groundwork for the remaining chapters. "Holistic Approaches to Preventing and Managing Alzheimer's Disease" is an invaluable and comprehensive resource for individuals, caregivers, healthcare professionals, and researchers seeking a deeper understanding of Alzheimer's disease and effective preventive strategies.

In Chapter 2, the author guides the reader through the concepts and methods of holistic health, defines holistic wellness, and discusses the relationship between integrative medicine and Alzheimer's disease. It also covers the mind-body connection and the critical role that nutrition plays in cognitive health, laying the groundwork for the holistic tactics that are covered in later chapters.

Chapters 3 to 8 meticulously examine specific holistic approaches. Chapter 3 emphasizes the impact of physical exercise on brain health, providing insights into suitable exercise types and personalized plans. Chapter 4 focuses on cognitive stimulation and mental health, incorporating brain training exercises, cognitive activities, and therapeutic interventions like music, art, meditation, and mindfulness. Chapter 5 investigates nutritional strategies, emphasizing the role of nutrition, superfoods, dietary patterns, and supplements in brain health. Chapter 6 addresses sleep and stress management, underscoring the importance of quality sleep, identifying sleep disorders, and exploring stress reduction techniques. Chapter 7 emphasizes the significance of social engagement, offering guidance on building connections and emotional support, while Chapter 8 delves into environmental factors and their impact on Alzheimer's risk, guiding readers in creating brain-healthy living environments and sustainable practices.

In Chapter 9, the book wraps up with helpful advice on how to incorporate holistic approaches into everyday life. It covers creating customized holistic plans, overcoming obstacles, and tracking advancement. In Chapter 10, real-world examples, expert interviews, and motivational stories reinforce the effectiveness of holistic approaches in managing and preventing Alzheimer's disease. To put it another way, this book acts as a lighthouse in the field, bridging the gap between theoretical knowledge and practical implementation, ultimately leading to a holistic and informed approach to Alzheimer's disease.

Overview

Alzheimer's disease (AD) is becoming more and more common, which presents a major challenge to global public health. This neurodegenerative disorder not only lowers the quality of life for individuals but also places a significant burden on healthcare systems and society at large. As research uncovers more and more of the complex factors that contribute to AD, prevention, and management of the disease must take a holistic approach. This comprehensive strategy addresses everything from genetic predispositions to lifestyle factors to promote cognitive health and reduce the impact of AD. This discussion explores the diverse aspects of holistic approaches and highlights their significance in AD prevention and management.

Context And Importance

Alzheimer's disease (AD) has a complex history that includes aging populations, genetic predispositions, and environmental factors. It is important to comprehend these factors to develop effective preventive measures and management strategies. Additionally, given the widespread impact AD has on individuals, families, and society, AD must be addressed comprehensively. By addressing the historical background and current challenges, researchers and healthcare professionals can pave the way for innovative and holistic approaches that go beyond conventional interventions.

The Book's Objective

An all-encompassing guide for researchers, healthcare professionals, and people affected by or worried about Alzheimer's disease (AD) is what a book on holistic approaches to the prevention and management of AD is supposed to do. It should bring together the most recent research findings, evidence-based practices, and holistic methodologies into one cohesive resource. It should also explain the various strategies and underlying principles so that readers can make well-informed decisions about AD prevention and management.

Intended Audience

This book attempts to bridge the gap between scientific knowledge and practical application by catering to the needs of diverse stakeholders, including researchers, healthcare practitioners, caregivers, policymakers, and individuals interested in promoting cognitive health. Whether the reader is a scientist seeking deeper insights into AD mechanisms or a caregiver looking for holistic strategies, the book strives to provide useful and approachable information.

Range And Restraints

The book covers a wide range of holistic approaches to AD, from dietary changes and lifestyle modifications to technology developments and community involvement. It aims to provide a holistic framework that takes into account the interaction of biological, psychological, and social factors. That being said, it is important to recognize the limitations that come with any comprehensive project: the book might not cover every aspect of AD, and new research could bring fresh insights. Furthermore, individual differences in how different holistic interventions work might make it difficult to create guidelines that apply to everyone.

Integrative Methods For Managing And Preventing Alzheimer's

A central component of a holistic strategy for the prevention and treatment of Alzheimer's disease is lifestyle modification. Studies show that certain lifestyle choices are strongly associated with the risk of developing AD. Regular exercise, eating a balanced diet high in antioxidants and omega-3 fatty acids, controlling stress, and participating in mentally stimulating activities are all important ways to support cognitive health.

Social interaction and participation in intellectually stimulating activities are also important. A holistic approach acknowledges the interdependence of these lifestyle factors and supports tailored interventions that cater to the individual's needs and preferences.

Comprehensive Method: Cognitive Excitation

Integrating cognitive stimulation into daily routines not only improves cognitive function but also promotes overall well-being. Holistic interventions in this domain recognize the value of lifelong learning and the potential benefits of staying mentally active throughout one's lifespan. Cognitive stimulation is a fundamental component of holistic approaches to AD.

This concept involves activities that challenge and engage the brain, promoting neuroplasticity and cognitive reserve. Cognitive stimulation encompasses a wide range of exercises, including puzzles, games, and learning new skills.

The goal is to keep the brain active and resilient against the neurodegenerative processes associated with AD.

Holistic Methodology: Dietary Measurements

Nutritional interventions are important in the prevention and treatment of Alzheimer's disease. A holistic approach to nutrition takes into account eating habits in general as well as specific dietary choices. Fruits and vegetables, which are high in antioxidants, are highlighted for their possible neuroprotective effects. Adding a Mediterranean or DASH (Dietary Approaches to Stop Hypertension) diet has also been shown to reduce the risk of AD. Holistic nutritional approaches also address issues like proper nutrient absorption and hydration.

Holistic Methodology: Mind-Body Techniques

Holistic interventions in the field of AD incorporate mind-body practices such as meditation, yoga, and tai chi, which have been practiced for centuries and are now recognized for their beneficial effects on mental and physical well-being. Studies have indicated that mind-body practices may have neuroprotective effects and support the maintenance of cognitive function. By combining these practices into an integrated approach, people can develop a harmonious and balanced relationship between their mind and body and promote a state of well-being that extends to their cognitive health.

Comprehensive Method: Technological Advancements

Technology offers a wide range of tools, from cognitive training apps to virtual reality experiences that stimulate the brain. Wearables and smart home technologies can help monitor and manage aspects of daily life, offering valuable insights into behavior patterns. The integration of technological innovations is a modern aspect of holistic approaches to AD. The holistic perspective on technology recognizes the potential for personalized and adaptive interventions, catering to individual needs and preferences.

However, while embracing technological advancements, it is important to consider ethical implications, data privacy, and accessibility to ensure that these innovations positively contribute to AD prevention and management.

Comprehensive Strategy: Community Involvement

Building dementia-friendly communities involves increasing awareness, lowering stigma, and creating environments that support individuals affected by AD. Holistic interventions in this domain extend beyond the individual and emphasize the collective responsibility of communities in promoting cognitive health. Initiatives like memory cafes, community education programs, and support groups contribute to a holistic ecosystem that addresses the diverse needs of individuals living with AD and their caregivers.

Community engagement is a crucial component of holistic approaches to AD, which recognize the social determinants of health and the impact of community support on cognitive well-being.

a holistic approach to preventing and managing Alzheimer's disease is a multifaceted endeavor that considers various interconnected factors.

The concepts discussed, including lifestyle modifications, cognitive stimulation, nutritional interventions, mind-body practices, technological innovations, and community engagement, collectively form a comprehensive framework. This holistic perspective recognizes the complexity of AD and emphasizes the importance of tailored interventions that address the unique characteristics of individuals. As research advances and our understanding of AD evolves, continued exploration and integration of holistic approaches will be crucial in developing effective strategies to mitigate the impact of this challenging neurodegenerative disorder. This book serves as a guide for those seeking a deeper understanding of holistic approaches, fostering collaboration and knowledge exchange among diverse stakeholders committed to the well-being of individuals affected by Alzheimer's disease.

CHAPTER ONE
UNDERSTANDING ALZHEIMER'S DISEASE

Alzheimer's disease is a neurodegenerative disorder that causes progressive cognitive decline, memory loss, and impaired functional abilities. After decades of research, a definitive cure for the disease is still elusive, so it is important to understand the disease in its entirety, starting with its definition and characteristics. The main indicator of Alzheimer's disease is the build-up of abnormal protein aggregates in the brain, such as tau tangles and beta-amyloid plaques, which disrupt neuronal communication and cause cognitive dysfunction.

Reasons And Danger Elements

The etiology of Alzheimer's disease is a result of a complex interplay between genetic, environmental, and lifestyle factors.

Genetics is involved, as certain gene mutations increase susceptibility, but environmental factors also have a significant impact. The risk of developing Alzheimer's disease has been associated with factors like diet, education level, and cardiovascular health. New research also suggests a possible link between chronic inflammation, insulin resistance, and the onset of the disease.

Alzheimer's Disease Stages

Alzheimer's disease progresses in several stages, each of which is distinguished by a different degree of cognitive decline. The first stage is frequently characterized by mild memory impairments; the following stages see a decline in language skills, reasoning, and problem-solving abilities; as the disease progresses, people experience severe memory loss and become unable to perform daily activities; in the final stages, communication becomes extremely difficult, and people may lose the ability to recognize loved ones. Knowledge of these stages is essential for developing interventions that target specific cognitive and functional impairments at different stages of the disease progression.

Current Methods Of Treatment

Alzheimer's disease is currently treated primarily with medications that aim to manage symptoms rather than provide a permanent cure. Memantine and cholinesterase inhibitors, for example, are medications that are used to temporarily slow down the progression of the disease and alleviate cognitive symptoms. Cognitive stimulation and behavioral therapies are examples of non-pharmacological interventions that are used to improve the quality of life for individuals with Alzheimer's disease. Despite their limitations, these treatments highlight the urgent need for new and more effective treatments.

The Requirement Of Holistic Methods

Given the shortcomings of existing treatments, there is a growing emphasis on holistic approaches to prevent and manage Alzheimer's disease. Holistic care takes into account the interdependence of different factors that impact health, such as physical, psychological, and social aspects. When it comes to Alzheimer's, a holistic approach addresses the individual's overall well-being in addition to cognitive symptoms.

This includes lifestyle changes, social interactions, nutritional interventions, and mental health support.

A balanced diet and regular exercise are effective in lowering the risk of Alzheimer's disease and delaying its progression. Brain health and cardiovascular health are closely related, and a diet high in antioxidants, omega-3 fatty acids, and other neuroprotective nutrients may help maintain cognitive function.

Holistic approaches also highlight the value of mental stimulation from games, puzzles, and lifelong learning to support cognitive resilience.

Maintaining meaningful social connections can improve emotional well-being and lessen the effects of cognitive decline. Programs that encourage community involvement, caregiver support groups, and interpersonal relationship-promoting interventions all contribute to a more thorough and successful approach to Alzheimer's care. Social engagement is crucial to the holistic care of individuals with Alzheimer's disease.

Nutritional therapies, such as customized meal plans and supplementation, are becoming more and more recognized as potential parts of integrative Alzheimer's care. Several nutrients, including omega-3 fatty acids and vitamins E and C, have been shown to have neuroprotective qualities. Dietary changes that address metabolic issues like insulin resistance may also improve cognitive function.

Considering the emotional toll that Alzheimer's takes on both the patient and the caregiver, mental health support is a crucial part of holistic care. Including psychotherapeutic interventions, counseling, and mindfulness practices can help reduce the stress, anxiety, and depression that come with the disease. These mental health components improve the patient's overall quality of life and foster a more supportive environment for caregivers.

the complexity of Alzheimer's disease necessitates a holistic approach that goes beyond traditional treatment modalities. Knowledge of the disease's definition, traits, causes, and phases serves as a basis for the development of all-encompassing interventions. Holistic approaches, which include dietary changes, social interactions, lifestyle adjustments, and mental health support, address the various facets of Alzheimer's and provide a more complex and successful approach to prevention and management. As research advances, incorporating these holistic ideas into standard Alzheimer's care has the potential to improve outcomes and the lives of those impacted by this difficult illness.

CHAPTER TWO
HOLISTIC PRINCIPLES AND APPROACHES

Adopting holistic principles can help individuals and healthcare professionals work towards a more comprehensive understanding and management of Alzheimer's disease. Holistic approaches to managing and preventing Alzheimer's disease emphasize the interconnectedness of various aspects of an individual's health—physical, mental, emotional, and social. This approach considers the whole person, recognizing that the mind and body are intricately linked, and aims to promote overall well-being rather than merely addressing isolated symptoms.

What Is Meant By Holistic Health?

Holistic health is a broad term that goes beyond the absence of illness or disease.

It is a state of total well-being that recognizes the interdependence of all aspects of life.

When it comes to managing and preventing Alzheimer's disease, holistic health highlights the significance of treating the person as a whole instead of just concentrating on cognitive symptoms. This more comprehensive viewpoint supports interventions that address lifestyle, emotional well-being, social connections, and environmental factors, all of which have an impact on cognitive health.

Holistic Approach To Well-Being

To promote a holistic sense of wellness, strategies for the prevention and management of Alzheimer's disease should go beyond pharmaceutical interventions and incorporate lifestyle modifications, emotional support, intellectual stimulation, and spiritual well-being.

The holistic model of wellness offers a framework for understanding health that goes beyond the traditional medical model.

It considers multiple dimensions, including physical, emotional, social, intellectual, and spiritual aspects of an individual's life.

Alzheimer's Disease And Integrative Medicine

When it comes to Alzheimer's disease, an integrative approach integrates evidence-based medical interventions with complementary therapies like acupuncture, massage, mindfulness, and nutritional counseling. By incorporating various modalities, integrative medicine aims to improve the overall well-being of individuals affected by Alzheimer's disease, addressing both the disease's symptoms and the larger aspects of their health. Integrative medicine emphasizes the importance of treating the whole person by combining conventional medical treatments with complementary and alternative therapies.

Mind-Body Link

The bidirectional relationship between mental and physical health is increasingly recognized as having a profound impact on overall well-being. Stress management, cognitive exercises, and mindfulness techniques are integral components of a holistic approach to Alzheimer's care.

By fostering a positive mind-body connection, individuals may experience improvements in cognitive function as well as enhanced emotional resilience and an overall improved quality of life. The mind-body connection is crucial to holistic approaches to preventing and managing Alzheimer's disease.

Nutrition's Significance For Cognitive Health

The impact of nutrition on cognitive health is well-established, and a holistic approach to managing and preventing Alzheimer's disease highlights the importance of a well-balanced diet. Specific dietary patterns, such as the Mediterranean diet, have been linked to a decreased risk of cognitive decline. Certain nutrients, such as vitamins, antioxidants, and omega-3 fatty acids, have specific roles in brain health. Holistic interventions take into account not only dietary recommendations but also the needs of each patient, taking into account factors like inflammation and gut health.

As a result, a holistic approach to the prevention and management of Alzheimer's disease entails embracing a comprehensive understanding of health and well-being. Healthcare professionals and individuals can develop more effective strategies for Alzheimer's prevention and management by integrating holistic principles, taking into account the mind-body connection, adopting a holistic model of wellness, investigating integrative medicine, and highlighting the significance of nutrition. This multifaceted approach acknowledges that cognitive health is influenced by a complex interplay of factors and encourages interventions that address the various facets of an individual's life.

CHAPTER THREE
FITNESS AND PREVENTION OF ALZHEIMER'S DISEASE

A key element of the integrative strategy for both preventing and treating Alzheimer's disease is physical exercise. Several studies have emphasized the beneficial effects of regular exercise on brain health, stressing its ability to slow cognitive deterioration and lower the risk of Alzheimer's. Physical activity has also been linked to several neuroprotective mechanisms, such as increased blood flow, decreased inflammation, and the stimulation of neurotrophic factors, which aid in the development and preservation of neurons.

Exercise's Effect On Brain Health

Exercise has a complex and multifaceted effect on brain health, involving complex physiological processes. Specifically, aerobic exercise has been associated with better cognitive function and a decreased risk of Alzheimer's. Consistent physical activity also improves cardiovascular health, which increases blood flow to the brain and supports optimal neuronal function. Exercise has also been shown to stimulate the release of neurotrophic factors, such as brain-derived neurotrophic factor (BDNF), which fosters the growth and survival of neurons. These neuroprotective effects reinforce the brain's overall resilience against age-related cognitive decline and neurodegenerative diseases like Alzheimer's.

Exercise Types That Are Good For Cognitive Function

Exercises that target different aspects of the brain have been shown to improve cognitive function. Aerobic exercises, like swimming, jogging, and brisk walking, have been studied extensively for their beneficial effects on cognitive health.

These exercises not only improve cardiovascular fitness but also encourage neuroplasticity, the brain's capacity to reorganize and adapt. Resistance training, which includes exercises like weightlifting, enhances muscle strength and physical well-being and indirectly influences cognitive health by lowering the risk of conditions that could exacerbate cognitive decline.

 Lastly, mind-body exercises, like yoga and tai chi, have been linked to stress reduction and enhanced mental clarity, both of which are factors that are linked to cognitive decline.

To optimize the benefits of exercise in the prevention of Alzheimer's disease, individualized exercise plans that are customized to each person's needs and abilities are necessary. Age, fitness level, and health conditions are just a few of the factors that must be considered when creating these plans. Working in conjunction with medical professionals, such as doctors and physical therapists, can help to guarantee that the exercise program is in line with the overall health goals of the individual and targets specific risk factors for Alzheimer's disease. Personalized plans may involve a mix of aerobic, resistance, and mind-body exercises that are carefully calibrated to offer a comprehensive approach to brain health.

Case Studies And Stories Of Triumph

Studying case studies and success stories provides a strong argument for the effectiveness of physical exercise in Alzheimer's prevention strategies. Many people have benefited from regular exercise in terms of cognitive function and overall well-being; these cases demonstrate the potential for improvement even in individuals who are at risk or in the early stages of the disease.

Success stories serve as a source of inspiration for those looking for practical ways to manage Alzheimer's disease; they also shed light on the various approaches and exercise modalities that have produced positive results, highlighting the need for tailored and comprehensive

physical exercise is a fundamental component of the integrated approach to both preventing and treating Alzheimer's disease. Research has shown that exercise has a positive impact on brain health, including increased blood flow, neurotrophic factor release, and neuroplasticity, which highlights its importance in reducing cognitive decline. Various forms of exercise, when combined into customized plans, enhance overall well-being. Positive outcomes achieved through regular exercise are demonstrated by case studies and success stories, which give hope and motivation to those who are at risk or who have been impacted by Alzheimer's.

CHAPTER FOUR
MENTAL HEALTH AND COGNITIVE STIMULATION

A holistic approach emphasizes the significance of maintaining cognitive function throughout the aging process. Cognitive stimulation involves a variety of activities designed to challenge and engage the brain, promoting neural plasticity and resilience. It involves exercises and interventions that aim to enhance memory, attention, problem-solving skills, and overall cognitive abilities. Cognitive stimulation plays a crucial role in preventing and managing Alzheimer's disease because it targets the cognitive functions affected by the condition.

Exercises For Brain Training

Engaging in regular brain training exercises has been linked to improved cognitive performance and may help to reduce the risk of cognitive decline. Brain training exercises are a cornerstone of cognitive stimulation in the prevention and management of Alzheimer's disease. They are specifically designed to target different cognitive functions and often involve activities like puzzles, memory games, and problem-solving tasks that challenge the brain and promote the formation of new neural connections. The concept is rooted in the idea of neuroplasticity, the brain's ability to reorganize itself by forming new neural connections throughout life.

Different Stages Of Cognitive Activities

Adapting cognitive activities to the various stages of Alzheimer's disease is critical to maximizing their effectiveness. Activities that promote memory, attention, and executive functions are especially helpful in the early stages, when cognitive decline may be mild. Activities may need to be modified as the disease advances to account for changing cognitive abilities.

In later stages, simpler tasks that emphasize emotional connection and sensory stimulation become crucial. The flexibility of cognitive activities guarantees that people with Alzheimer's disease at different stages can continue to benefit from cognitive stimulation, which adds to a more comprehensive and individualized approach to care.

Art Therapy And Music

Both music therapy and art therapy have gained recognition as important elements of holistic approaches to the prevention and management of Alzheimer's disease. These creative interventions draw on emotional and aesthetic dimensions, offering avenues for expression and engagement. Research has demonstrated that music therapy, which involves listening to or making music, can elicit emotional responses, stimulate memories, and improve communication in individuals with Alzheimer's disease. Art therapy, which includes activities like painting, drawing, and crafting, offers a non-verbal outlet for self-expression. When verbal abilities are compromised, both modalities offer a means of connection and communication, which improves the overall well-being of individuals with Alzheimer's disease.

Mindfulness And Meditation Techniques

By addressing the psychological and emotional aspects of the disease, meditation, and mindfulness practices play a significant role in the holistic management of Alzheimer's disease. Mindfulness-based interventions, like deep breathing exercises and meditation, have been shown to positively impact cognitive function and emotional well-being. By promoting a sense of calm and focus, these practices may contribute to improved quality of life for individuals with Alzheimer's and their caregivers. Integrating meditation and mindfulness into care plans adds a dimension of holistic support, acknowledging the psychological and emotional aspects of the condition.

a comprehensive care strategy that recognizes the various needs of individuals at different stages of the disease and promotes both cognitive and emotional well-being benefits from a holistic approach that emphasizes cognitive stimulation and mental health interventions. Brain training exercises, customized cognitive activities, music and art therapy, as well as meditation and mindfulness practices, all contribute to this multifaceted approach. As research in this area advances, more investigation into these concepts and their incorporation into personalized care plans holds promise for improving the overall quality of life for those affected by Alzheimer's disease.

CHAPTER FIVE
DIETARY APPROACHES TO MAINTAIN BRAIN HEALTH

A balanced and nutrient-rich diet is essential for maintaining brain health and preventing cognitive decline. Vital nutrients like omega-3 fatty acids, antioxidants, vitamins, and minerals are essential components that support optimal brain function. For example, omega-3 fatty acids found in fish oil have been linked to improved cognitive performance and a decreased risk of developing neurodegenerative diseases. Research on the relationship between nutrition and cognitive function is crucial to holistic approaches to preventing and managing Alzheimer's disease.

Recently, there has been a lot of talk about superfoods for brain health. These are nutrient-dense foods that are high in antioxidants, vitamins, and minerals that support overall health, including cognitive health.

Superfoods like dark leafy greens, avocados, walnuts, and blueberries are thought to have neuroprotective effects, which may reduce the risk of Alzheimer's disease. Understanding the molecular mechanisms by which these superfoods interact with the brain is essential to developing their therapeutic potential.

Dietary habits are critical to preventing Alzheimer's disease. Following a Mediterranean or DASH (Dietary Approaches to Stop Hypertension) diet has been linked to a decreased risk of cognitive decline and Alzheimer's disease. These diets emphasize fruits, vegetables, whole grains, lean proteins, and healthy fats while reducing the intake of processed foods, sugars, and saturated fats. These dietary habits have a complex cumulative effect on brain health, affecting variables like oxidative stress, inflammation, and vascular function.

Another way to support cognitive health is with supplements and vitamins. Although getting nutrients from a well-balanced diet is ideal, some supplements may have extra benefits.

For example, vitamin E, which has been shown to have antioxidant properties, may be able to slow cognitive decline. However, it is important to use supplements sparingly because taking too much of some vitamins can have negative effects.

 Research is still being done to determine the best dosage and combinations of supplements that may protect neurons without harming them.

The complex interactions between particular nutrients, superfoods, dietary patterns, and supplements highlight the difficulty of preserving cognitive function. More research is required to elucidate the mechanisms underlying the influence of nutrition on brain health and to develop evidence-based guidelines for successful preventive strategies. In summary, nutritional strategies for brain health are essential parts of holistic approaches to preventing and managing Alzheimer's disease.

Engaging In Exercise And Improving Cognitive Function

The two main pillars of the integrative strategy for Alzheimer's disease prevention and management are physical exercise and cognitive stimulation. Studies have shown that regular physical activity has a significant impact on brain health.

Aerobic exercises, like walking, jogging, or swimming, have been linked to a lower risk of Alzheimer's disease and cognitive decline.

The mechanisms by which physical activity provides neuroprotective effects on the brain include increased blood flow, the release of neurotrophic factors, and enhanced synaptic plasticity.

Apart from physical exercise, cognitive stimulation is essential for preserving cognitive function and averting Alzheimer's disease. Brain-taxing activities like games, puzzles, and learning new skills encourage cognitive reserve, or the brain's capacity to tolerate pathology. Cognitive stimulation strengthens neural connections, encourages neuroplasticity, and may postpone the onset of cognitive decline. Moreover, lifelong participation in intellectually stimulating activities may help accumulate a cognitive reserve that acts as a protective shield against the consequences of neurodegenerative processes.

It has been shown that the combination of physical activity and cognitive stimulation is especially effective in promoting brain health. Research indicates that a combined strategy that incorporates both components may have synergistic effects in lowering the risk of Alzheimer's disease. For example, physical and mental activities like dancing or specific sports may offer greater benefits than isolated interventions. Knowledge of the best kind, amount, and duration of physical activity as well as the variety and complexity of cognitive stimulation is essential for creating customized preventive strategies.

Neurotrophic factors, neurogenesis, neuroinflammation, and modulation of different neurotransmitter systems are among the complex and multifaceted potential mechanisms that link physical activity and cognitive stimulation to the prevention of Alzheimer's disease.

More research is required to clarify these mechanisms and determine the most effective interventions for various populations and stages of life.

The combination of physical activity and cognitive stimulation offers a multimodal strategy to improve brain health and lower the risk of cognitive decline. Personalized and sustainable interventions that take into account individual preferences, capacities, and lifestyles are crucial for the successful implementation of these strategies on a larger scale. In conclusion, physical activity and cognitive stimulation are essential components of holistic approaches to Alzheimer's prevention and management.

Stress Reduction And Sleep Hygiene

In holistic approaches to cognitive health, the importance of stress management and sleep hygiene in preventing and managing Alzheimer's disease is becoming more widely acknowledged. Good sleep is critical for brain health and cognitive functions; it is important for memory consolidation, synaptic plasticity, and the removal of toxins from the brain, including beta-amyloid, a protein linked to Alzheimer's disease. Sleep disturbances, like insomnia or sleep apnea, have been linked to a higher risk of cognitive decline.

Another factor that affects cognitive health and may play a role in the development of Alzheimer's disease is stress, both acute and chronic. Prolonged stress exposure can cause the hypothalamic-pituitary-adrenal (HPA) axis to dysregulate, which raises cortisol levels. Chronically high cortisol is linked to inflammation, reduced neurogenesis, and impaired hippocampal function—all of which are linked to cognitive decline and neurodegenerative diseases.

Practices that help mitigate the physiological effects of stress and promote emotional well-being include mindfulness meditation, yoga, and relaxation techniques. Mindfulness-based interventions in particular have shown promise in reducing symptoms of anxiety and depression, which are common contributors to chronic stress. These and other effective stress management strategies have been shown to positively impact brain health.

There is a reciprocal relationship between stress, sleep hygiene, and Alzheimer's disease: chronic stress can negatively impact sleep quality, and disrupted sleep patterns can exacerbate stress. To promote cognitive health, a comprehensive approach that addresses stress management and sleep hygiene must be put into practice. Personalized interventions that take into account each person's unique sleep needs, lifestyle factors, and stressors are critical to the success of these strategies.

Current research focuses on the molecular and cellular mechanisms that connect stress, sleep, and Alzheimer's disease. Developing targeted interventions requires an understanding of how sleep and stress affect processes like neuroinflammation, synaptic plasticity, and the build-up of pathological proteins. Additionally, exploring potential synergies between stress management, sleep hygiene, and other preventive measures like physical activity and nutrition is crucial for comprehensive Alzheimer's prevention.

holistic approaches to the prevention and management of Alzheimer's disease must prioritize good sleep hygiene and effective stress management. These lifestyle choices are critical for maintaining cognitive health and lowering the risk of neurodegenerative diseases, and they also contribute to general well-being.

Creating public health campaigns that emphasize the value of sleep and stress management and offering easily accessible resources for putting these strategies into practice is crucial for promoting brain health in a variety of populations.

CHAPTER SIX
MANAGING STRESS AND SLEEP

The importance of quality sleep in preventing and managing Alzheimer's disease cannot be overstated. Quality sleep is defined as having enough duration, continuity, and depth, which helps to restore and consolidate memory and cognitive functions. Research indicates that inadequate or disrupted sleep may have a significant impact on brain health and increase the risk of developing neurodegenerative conditions like Alzheimer's disease. It is crucial to comprehend the complex relationship between sleep and cognitive health to develop holistic approaches to address Alzheimer's risk.

Several sleep disorders are significant risk factors for Alzheimer's disease. Disorders such as insomnia, sleep apnea, and restless leg syndrome, for example, have been associated with a higher risk of cognitive decline and the emergence of neurodegenerative disorders. Developing targeted prevention and management strategies for Alzheimer's disease requires an understanding of the mechanisms by which these sleep disorders contribute to the disease. Additionally, investigating the reciprocal relationship between sleep disturbances and Alzheimer's pathology offers important insights into potential intervention points.

Stress, a ubiquitous feature of contemporary life, has been found to have a substantial impact on cognitive health and may even accelerate the development of Alzheimer's disease.

Prolonged stress can cause the hypothalamic-pituitary-adrenal (HPA) axis to become dysregulated, releasing excessive cortisol that may have deleterious effects on the structure and function of the brain. By comprehending the complex mechanisms by which stress affects cognitive health, comprehensive interventions can be developed.

The fact that stress is a modifiable risk factor for Alzheimer's emphasizes the significance of integrating stress management into holistic approaches for prevention and management.

Relaxation techniques are essential when it comes to treating stress as a risk factor for Alzheimer's. Methods like progressive muscle relaxation, deep breathing exercises, and mindfulness meditation have demonstrated the potential to reduce the physiological and psychological effects of stress. These approaches not only foster a feeling of peace and well-being but also have the potential to positively impact brain health. By integrating these relaxation techniques into lifestyle interventions, they become more feasible and long-lasting, providing individuals with useful tools to manage stress and possibly lower their risk of Alzheimer's disease.

The integration of relaxation techniques into holistic approaches offers individuals practical tools to mitigate stress and potentially lower their risk of Alzheimer's disease.

Quality sleep is fundamental, with sleep disorders posing as potential risk factors for Alzheimer's. Stress, a pervasive and modifiable factor, significantly influences cognitive health, emphasizing the need for stress management strategies. Researchers and healthcare professionals can formulate more effective strategies for preventing and managing Alzheimer's disease by thoroughly understanding the intricate interplay between sleep, stress, and cognitive health.

CHAPTER SEVEN
EMOTIONAL HEALTH AND SOCIAL ENGAGEMENT

A comprehensive strategy for preventing and managing Alzheimer's disease must address social isolation as a significant risk factor. Interventions should emphasize social engagement among individuals, participation in social activities, and fostering connections within communities. Social isolation and cognitive decline are closely related, especially in the context of Alzheimer's disease. Research indicates that individuals who experience social isolation may be at a higher risk of cognitive decline and an increased likelihood of developing Alzheimer's. This phenomenon is attributed to the lack of cognitive stimulation and mental activity that social interactions provide.

A key component of the holistic approach to Alzheimer's prevention and management is the development of strong social networks, which have been demonstrated to have a protective effect on cognitive function, functioning as a buffer against the deleterious effects of cognitive decline. Regular social interactions and meaningful relationships also support cognitive reserve, the brain's capacity to function normally in the face of injury.

As such, efforts should be focused on improving social support networks, creating opportunities for socialization, and encouraging community engagement. These can be accomplished through community-based programs, support groups, and initiatives that promote social interaction among individuals at risk of or already managing Alzheimer's.

A holistic approach should include strategies for emotional support, such as counseling services, support groups, and educational opportunities. Emotional support is essential for the well-being of both individuals with Alzheimer's disease and their caregivers. The emotional impact of Alzheimer's disease can be overwhelming, resulting in increased stress, anxiety, and depression. Providing emotional support involves creating an environment that is conducive to open communication, empathy, and understanding. Caregivers, in particular, require adequate emotional support to cope with the challenges associated with caregiving.

Community engagement initiatives, like dementia-friendly neighborhoods, help raise awareness and reduce the stigma surrounding Alzheimer's disease, fostering a supportive environment for affected individuals. Communities can serve as a valuable source of support, offering resources and programs that cater to the specific needs of individuals with Alzheimer's and their caregivers. Communities can be a valuable source of support, offering resources and programs that cater to the needs of individuals with Alzheimer's and their caregivers.

In summary, the multifaceted approach highlights the significance of social engagement and emotional well-being in the prevention and management of Alzheimer's disease. Important components of this approach include addressing social isolation, fostering strong social connections, offering emotional support, and making use of community resources and programs. By putting into practice comprehensive strategies that take into account the social and emotional aspects of individuals affected by Alzheimer's disease, we can improve their overall well-being and potentially lessen the disease's impact on cognitive function.

CHAPTER EIGHT
ENVIRONMENTAL ASPECTS AND ALZHEIMER'S RISK

Alzheimer's disease is a complex neurodegenerative disease with a multifactorial etiology that includes genetic, lifestyle, and environmental factors. When investigating the environmental factors that influence the risk of Alzheimer's disease, it is critical to examine the role of environmental toxins.

Certain environmental toxins have been associated with a higher risk of Alzheimer's disease. For example, exposure to heavy metals like lead and mercury, as well as air pollutants like particulate matter, has been linked to cognitive decline and an increased risk of Alzheimer's disease. Studies indicate that these toxins may contribute to the buildup of tau tangles and amyloid-beta plaques, two hallmark pathological features of Alzheimer's disease.

Therefore, it is important to comprehend and mitigate the impact of environmental toxins.

Building A Living Space That Is Brain-Healthy

Establishing a brain-healthy living environment entails making lifestyle decisions that support cognitive well-being. These decisions touch on a variety of areas of daily life, such as nutrition, physical exercise, and mental stimulation.

Diet is a critical component of brain health; a diet high in antioxidants, omega-3 fatty acids, and other essential nutrients has been linked to a decreased risk of Alzheimer's disease. Physical exercise regularly has also been linked to cognitive benefits, lowering the risk of cognitive decline and promoting overall brain health. Mental stimulation, which can be achieved through activities like reading, puzzles, and social interaction, can also support cognitive resilience. As a result, developing a brain-healthy living environment

Long-Term Strategies For Mental Well-Being:

Embracing sustainable practices for cognitive wellness is essential to the pursuit of a holistic approach to Alzheimer's prevention and management. Sustainable practices go beyond individual lifestyle decisions to take into account societal and environmental factors.

Taking a sustainable approach entails advocating for practices that benefit the individual's cognitive health as well as the larger ecosystem.

For example, supporting green spaces in urban planning can improve mental health and provide areas for physical activity. Additionally, sustainable farming practices that minimize exposure to potentially neurotoxic pesticides contribute to a cleaner environment.

Embracing these sustainable practices into daily life not only fosters cognitive wellness

All things considered, recognizing the impact of environmental toxins, developing brain-healthy living environments, and adopting sustainable practices for cognitive wellness are important steps toward understanding and addressing environmental factors in the context of Alzheimer's disease risk.

This all-encompassing approach acknowledges the complex interplay between individual lifestyle choices, environmental exposures, and societal considerations, and by taking these factors into account as a whole, we can develop effective strategies to prevent and manage Alzheimer's disease, thereby moving towards a more holistic and integrative paradigm in the field of cognitive health.

CHAPTER NINE
INCLUDING HOLISTIC APPROACHES IN EVERYDAY LIFE

The pursuit of preventing and managing Alzheimer's disease necessitates the integration of holistic approaches into daily life.

Holistic health emphasizes the interconnectedness of mind, body, and spirit, acknowledging that an individual's well-being is influenced by various factors.

Adopting a holistic lifestyle entails addressing not only the physical aspects of health but also mental, emotional, and social dimensions; it recognizes the importance of a balanced and harmonious existence. Integrating stress management techniques, a nutritious diet, regular physical exercise, and regular physical exercise are essential elements of holistic living. Completing puzzles and mental exercises are examples of activities that promote cognitive function and are integral parts of a holistic lifestyle.

Creating A Customized Comprehensive Strategy

Personalized plans may combine cognitive exercises, dietary modifications, stress reduction techniques, and targeted physical activities. Integrating alternative therapies, such as mindfulness meditation and aromatherapy, can also be considered based on an individual's preferences and responses. By recognizing and addressing specific risk factors and preferences, a personalized holistic plan becomes a powerful tool in promoting overall well-being and mitigating the effects of Alzheimer's disease. To develop a personalized holistic plan for Alzheimer's prevention and management, it is important to understand that each person's circumstances are unique.

Overcoming Obstacles And Difficulties

While there are many advantages to using holistic approaches for Alzheimer's prevention and management, people may run into several obstacles when putting these strategies into practice. These obstacles can include a lack of awareness, financial constraints, and cultural factors. Overcoming these obstacles calls for a multifaceted approach; financial barriers can be addressed through community resources and affordable health programs; knowledge-related barriers can be addressed by educating the public about the importance of holistic approaches through educational campaigns and community outreach; and cultural considerations must be taken into account when designing holistic plans to respect diverse beliefs and practices.

Tracking Development And Modifying Approaches

The implementation of a holistic approach to the prevention and management of Alzheimer's disease requires an ongoing process of monitoring progress and making adjustments to strategies.

To assess the efficacy of implemented holistic plans, regular assessments of cognitive function, emotional well-being, and overall health are necessary. Assessments may include cognitive tests, mood assessments, and physical health evaluations. By tracking changes over time, individuals and healthcare professionals can identify potential challenges or areas of improvement. Flexibility is essential when making adjustments to holistic strategies because individual responses may vary. Adapting plans based on ongoing assessments guarantees that interventions stay relevant and effective.

a comprehensive strategy for preventing and managing Alzheimer's disease involves incorporating these fundamental ideas into everyday life. Other crucial elements of this all-encompassing approach include creating a customized holistic plan based on each person's unique needs, overcoming obstacles, and continuously assessing the disease's progress, and making necessary adjustments to strategies.

By adopting holistic practices that take into account the interconnected aspects of well-being, people can maximize their chances of preserving cognitive health and lowering their risk of Alzheimer's disease.

CHAPTER TEN
CASE STUDIES AND TRIUMPHS

Case studies and success stories are essential for shedding light on the effectiveness of holistic approaches in the prevention and management of Alzheimer's disease. By carefully analyzing individual cases, researchers and practitioners can learn about the various strategies people use to either manage the disease or delay cognitive decline. Case studies are a great way to gather information for scientific analysis and can also serve as a source of inspiration for professionals and the general public. By analyzing the lifestyle, eating habits, cognitive activities, and general well-being of those who have successfully applied holistic approaches, patterns, and best practices can be found that help prevent and manage Alzheimer's disease.

Examples Of Holistic Approaches In The Real World

Empirical examples of holistic approaches provide concrete proof of the influence that lifestyle adjustments can have on the prevention and management of Alzheimer's disease.

These examples explore the lives of people who have embraced comprehensive strategies, such as regular exercise, dietary adjustments, cognitive stimulation, and social engagement.

By analyzing these real-life scenarios, researchers can pinpoint the precise factors that lead to successful outcomes. This investigation not only clarifies the complex nature of Alzheimer's prevention but also highlights the significance of

tailored, holistic interventions. Knowing the subtleties of how people incorporate these approaches into their daily lives offers a nuanced perspective for both practitioners and researchers.

Conversations With Subject Matter Experts

Experts in the field can provide in-depth explanations of the biological mechanisms involved, share the most recent research findings, and offer practical advice based on their professional experience. Interviews with neuroscientists, geriatricians, nutritionists, and other specialists allow for a nuanced exploration of the scientific underpinnings and practical applications of holistic strategies. These interviews serve as a bridge between scientific knowledge and real-world application, providing a well-rounded perspective that informs healthcare professionals and the general public about the significance of holistic approaches.

Motivating Narratives Of Alzheimer's Disease Prevention And Handling

Inspirational stories of people who have effectively prevented or managed Alzheimer's disease through holistic approaches are a powerful source of motivation for those who are currently dealing with the disease or those who are looking to proactively adopt preventative measures.

These stories are human and highlight the struggles faced by individuals and their families as well as the victories attained through determination and lifestyle changes.

Despite the data and expert opinions, these stories evoke strong emotions because they highlight the resilience and successes of those who have walked this path, which helps to foster a sense of hope, empowerment, and belief in the efficacy of holistic approaches in the face of Alzheimer's disease.

SUMMARY

To fully understand this complex condition, it is important to explore holistic approaches to managing and preventing Alzheimer's disease through case studies, real-world examples, expert interviews, and inspiring stories. The multifaceted nature of Alzheimer's necessitates a holistic perspective that takes into account lifestyle, nutrition, cognitive activities, and social engagement. Case studies and success stories offer concrete evidence of the effectiveness of holistic interventions, while expert interviews provide a deeper understanding of the scientific foundations. Lastly, inspiring stories infuse the discourse with a sense of hope and motivation while highlighting the potential for positive outcomes through proactive and comprehensive strategies.

Summary Of Holistic Methods

This overview of holistic approaches highlights the need for a multimodal and individualized approach to treating Alzheimer's disease. Lifestyle changes, such as regular exercise, a healthy diet, mental stimulation, and social interaction, all contribute to brain health and resilience.

These factors work together to create an environment that can either prevent or delay the onset of Alzheimer's disease.

Additionally, understanding the complex interactions between genetics, environmental factors, and lifestyle choices highlights the significance of individualized interventions. Finally, this overview serves as a reminder that holistic approaches are not a one-size-fits-all solution but rather a dynamic and adaptive framework that takes into account the uniqueness of each person's journey.

Optimism For The Future

While Alzheimer's disease presents many challenges, the investigation of holistic approaches offers hope for the future. The body of evidence from case studies, real-world examples, expert interviews, and motivational stories indicates that proactive lifestyle choices can impact the trajectory of the disease significantly.

Research advancements and an increasing recognition of the significance of holistic interventions add to the optimism surrounding the prevention and management of Alzheimer's disease. This optimism is based on the empowerment of individuals to take charge of their health and well-being as well as on scientific understanding. Looking ahead, the possibility of additional breakthroughs in holistic approaches provides a ray of hope for those impacted by or at risk for the disease.

Motivation For Peruses

Last but not least, this examination of holistic approaches to managing and preventing Alzheimer's is meant to inspire readers to take proactive measures toward brain health.

 The abundance of knowledge offered, bolstered by case studies, real-life examples, professional insights, and motivational tales, highlights the agency people have in molding their cognitive well-being. Each person's journey to managing or preventing Alzheimer's is different, and although obstacles may occur, the evidence presented here shows the potential for positive outcomes through holistic interventions. As readers set out on their paths toward brain health, this encouragement acts as a reminder that wise decisions and holistic approaches can clear the way for a better and more resilient future, not only for I